Networking: 42 Keys to Career Growth- Communication Skills, Building Relationships, Influence

Brett Longer

TABLE OF CONTENTS

INTRODUCTION

Thank you and congratulations for downloading the book, *Networking: 42 Keys to Career Growth- Communication Skills, Build Relationships, Influence."* The old saying of "It's not what you know, it's who you know" holds true today just as it did before. With jobs being more competitive, with a greater gap in qualifications and the need for experience for the younger folks, being very good at networking is essential to career gains.

My philosophy and hope in this book is to help you get the job even before there is a job. *Networking: 42 Keys* contains proven steps and strategies on how to help you get to the "point of no return." "The point of no return" is the space where they like you; they trust you and they want to work with you so much that the influence is almost on autopilot. I believe that this guide will lead you to the career growth you want and provide you with the tools to have the confidence and charm you need to win almost everyone you meet.

This book is meant to leave you with the most proven and studied ways to communicating clearly, confidently, and with a purpose. Networking is a tool that far too many just do not focus on and even fewer people master. It is a tool, when done right, that is just too powerful to ignore. The book should leave you with a greater understanding on how to gain trust and influence. Thanks again for downloading this book, I hope you enjoy it! Let's get started!

CHAPTER 1

WHAT IS NETWORKING?

If you want to have a flourishing career, then learning about networking can help you a lot. Networking has become an invaluable tool for people who are looking for ways to find opportunities and gather the right people to achieve massive goals. For this reason, it has become important for people to connect with each other, in one way or another.

If you are new to networking, then the best way for you to start is to go to networking events and find ways to socialize with people who may have the same goals and interests as yours. Networking events have a lot of things in store for those who are looking to expand their market and open a whole lot of opportunities. If you are looking for job or market leads, great business partners, or backers, then joining events and associations will work to your advantage

The People you will Find in Networking Events

Before you keep your hopes up and think that you are going to land massive career opportunities once you connect with the right people, hold that thought. If you are networking for the sake of raking in more profits the moment you get a business card, then you are doing this whole thing wrong.

Contrary to the popular belief that networking is as easy as shaking hands can get, the entire process is actually tough. That means to say that you will need to invest months, or even years, of your time in order for you to get something out of networking. The reason is simple – you simply do not walk into a room and get someone to hire you or give you a gig. You have to show a prospective employer or a partner that you are worth their time.

A lot of people who attend, or have attended, networking events find that these meet-ups are unnecessary and are only a waste of time and money. These are the people who are not able to find solid leads about how they are going to get the things that they want from those whom they met on an event. Apparently, these people are those who are only interested on telling others to give them what they want. They are those who do not want to take risks and build relationships first. With that said, it is safe to assume that they are the type of networkers who count their chickens before the eggs hatched. Give them a few years and they are likely to burn the bridges that they have made.

There are some people who leave these events happily, with a business card on their hands. These people know that they will be meeting those whom they have been introduced to, and that they will be willing to go the miles in order to have a strong relationship with them. If you are one of these people, then you may have found the secret ingredient of networking.

Why do people feel that networking does not work for them, and that it is futile to go out there to meet people? The reason is simple – they do not know how to network in the first place.

Why Networking is Better than Hiring or Applying?

Most of the people who have given up on networking think that they will be able to build their own empire without having to rely on anyone. However, those who truly grasp how networking works will beg to disagree. While a man can be successful and rich on his own, a person will only be able to achieve genuine stability with a little help from friends.

If you do think that you are better off scouting for a better-paying job or using your resources to hire the best employees out there, then think again. An employer may fire you, and employees may leave you for much greener pastures, but friends will never desert you.

Once you are able to connect to a person and turn him into an ally, all you need to do is to protect and nourish that relationship. What you will get in return is support in all things that you do, even if you change your branding or switch careers. Once you manage your networks well and encourage healthy competition and camaraderie with everyone that you are connected to, you successfully enable everyone to let each other peacefully coexist in a congested market. That means that even though you are connected to competition, both of you will still be able to thrive.

If you wonder what makes businesses and celebrities become extremely successful in this age where people have too much of everything, then you will realize that the secret ingredient to their wealth is their network. Your network allows you to market yourself without having to spend anything, just as long as you keep them in the loop. Your network will also provide you with a steady supply of niche audience who will support every kind of product that you would realize, and should you need any help in production, you will also be getting a steady source of suppliers. What's in it for them? Your friendship, of course.

Instead of living in a dog-eat-dog world, it is better to be a part of a pack. When you think of networking this way, you will realize how valuable other people are, no matter what field they are in.

Why Do Some People Fail in Networking?

People have always made it a point to meet other people, but they do not know how to maintain their connection with these newfound friends. The reason is simple – most people think about themselves, and because of that, they only think of how their network will be able to help them.

However, networking works differently. Instead of thinking how the people whom you just met will be able to help you get your dream job, you need to invest on them first. With that said, you need to focus on how they will find you helpful, instead of the other way around.

The key to networking is to start doing it even before you need it to work for you. You need to make sturdy bridges first before you even cross them, and because of that, you need to have a plan on how you are going to have solid connections with the people whom you have met when it is time to cash in your efforts. That would mean spending time to build the trust and respect that people have for you before you make huge demands or requests.

Keep in mind that building networks is just like building relationships – in order for them to work well and for them to last, you will need to nurture them first. Don't worry much about what you are going to get in return and when you are going to expect a payback. You will be reaping the fruits of your labor in no time at all, and you are going to be rewarded with results faster than you expect to receive them.

CHAPTER 2

KEYS 1- 10: MAKE A GOOD IMPRESSION

It's been said "first impressions last". Though you may have probably heard this a million times, it cannot be denied how this saying holds so much truth in our everyday interactions.

In your journey towards career growth and success, how you meet people for the first time determines how they will respond to and remember you. The way you leave a good first impression is the beginning of your relationship with others, and if you want to make a lasting and positive relationship, then it makes sense for you to spend time to think on what a person should remember the first time you meet.

Why First Impressions Last

There are many times when you have probably thought about the possibility of making it up on a second meeting, especially when you made a terrible introduction of yourself to someone you just met. You probably have met the best employer there is, but you did not have time to prepare yourself well for an interview. You may have met the best candidate to be your business partner, but you accidentally became dismissive when you first met. Is there any chance that you can take a second chance in order to gain their esteem?

Psychology says that while it may be possible, it will be extremely difficult to change first impressions. The reason is that since people associate particular incidents to the people they meet, and once an association has been done, it almost does not go away. First impressions are actually created at a fraction of a second, and people have always believed that the perception that they initially have of another person is more accurate than the succeeding impressions that that person may exhibit in the future.

Just think of this: imagine having bit by a dog as a child while walking home from school – it would almost be impossible for you to trust another stray dog to not hurt you, should you see one. That goes the same when you meet a person who strikes you as irresponsible or annoying. The chances of you desiring to work with such person would be zero, unless that person strives to win your esteem back. That, of course, will take a long time. One also needs to be in a similar situation again, and the experience should be rewarding.

Great Impressions Make Associations

Since what people remember the most is the way they met you, they will most likely hold on to that memory for a long time. With that said, they are also very likely to be forgiving if you make a few slips in the future. If you make succeeding meetings positive as well, then that would reinforce the great impression that they have of you.

So what actually makes up a good first impression? Dale Carnegie, author of the bestseller, How to Win Friends and Influence People, says that the only way to make a good impression is to be genuinely interested in others. People, by nature, are good judges of character – contrary to popular belief, it is almost impossible for a person to make it through a first meeting wearing a disguise or a well-rehearsed character. That means that people normally sense it when others are not being genuine with how they are making a relationship with them. It almost means that "judging a book by its cover" actually works – when you have doubts about the sincerity of the person that you have just met, then that gut feel really does have a bearing.

The main reason why humans behave this way is that like most living creatures in this planet, they normally want to connect and build future relationships with others who hold the promise of protecting their survival. People bond well with their kin or the ones who belong to their community because they have the same means of making it through daily struggles. When you have a firm belief that a person does not threaten you and that he is going to enrich your experience in more ways than one, then you are compelled to create a positive relationship during your first meeting. The reverse also holds true, and even when a person tries to change the initial impression that he made you have, the unpleasant memory of your initial meeting would still stick.

Ways to Make a Good First Impression

Is there any way for you to avoid blunders when you make your first impression? The key to making that initial impact positive and memorable is preparation. There are many ways for you to anticipate what a person will probably like in the people that he meets. For example, if you are going to meet a prospective employer through an initial interview, then it makes sense that you appear as a true professional. You will never want to appear with a disheveled hair, inappropriate attire, or unprepared to answer questions. You want to appear as the professional that you really are. By embodying a personality that many people find desirable when you first meet them, then you are on your way to creating a lasting network with them.

Here are the first ten networking keys that will help you make a good, lasting impression on prospective colleagues, clients, employers, and networks.

1 Wear a smile

The moment you enter the room, people are already sizing you up. This is often done subconsciously, sometimes intentionally. In all your interactions, it is a no-brainer practice to wear a smile and evoke a pleasant attitude. Smiling is the first step in giving off a good impression, building rapport, and setting the tone.

Smiling means being genuine. Nobody wants to meet someone with a fake smile masking a dull attitude. Your smile will come from within. To give off an authentic smile, you must first be genuinely interested in the person you are meeting. If you're in a gloomy mood or a nervous state, try to calm yourself down by taking a few deep breaths. This can go a long way in helping you be less focused on yourself and be diverted to the person you are meeting, thus making it easier to flash a real smile and a pleasant vibe.

Also keep in mind that when you are ready to walk into the room filled with people whom you want to build networks with, you would want to make them feel that you are interested in them, and not the other way around. You can make them feel that by thinking about how you can make them feel comfortable around you. Once you have that mindset, everything becomes automatic – you will immediately be flashing a welcoming smile the moment you enter the room.

2 Give a firm handshake

Many people know how to give off a welcoming smile, but are clueless when it comes to the impression they make from their feeble handshakes. Partner that charming smile with an equally charming grip. Handshakes symbolize your first physical contact with someone, and a firm handshake exudes a no-nonsense, determined, and strong individual.

Of course, your grip shouldn't be too firm that it will crush the other person's bones, but don't make it too weak and lifeless either.

Handshakes are very important when you introduce yourself to people with different cultural backgrounds. You do not have to wait for the other person to extend his hands into a handshake. Make sure that you offer yours first. By making this gesture, you are making the impression that you are confident and that you are willing to engage the other person into a more meaningful and enriching exchange.

3 Posture is everything

When making a good impression, it is imperative to have good posture. This means donning a straight back, a leveled chin (not too high and not drooping), open shoulders, and a gait that is a balance between modest and strong.

Good posture is not only an indication of confidence, but also of dependability. Most people immediately think that a person who can hold his posture is someone who will never have a problem with his communication skills and is willing to exert effort to make things work well. By making that impression, a person with a good posture also piques the interest of the person that he is meeting for the first time.

Posture is also a body language that shows how interested you are in another person. By assuming a confident but welcoming posture, you are sending the signal that you did not only walk into the room with self-esteem, but you are also very eager to meet other people. Without even having to speak, you are sending the impression to everyone that can see you at the corner of your eye that you are in the room to mingle with people with genuine interest in them.

When it comes to posture, it is best not to go extreme. Do not be too rigid, and do not be too loose and laidback either. Remember to evoke a strong persona while showing that you are relaxed and open.

4 Greetings

Many people have forgotten how to say proper greetings. Saying "hi" is often the first thing that comes out of everyone's mouths, but in more formal settings, it is best to say "good morning", "good afternoon", or "good evening" first. Saying these greetings before the actual conversation shows how well mannered and pleasant you are. After all, such greetings are meant to convey positivity and amiability.

Asking "how do you do" or "how are you" are also no-fail greetings. These show that you are interested in the other person. It is always nice to hear someone ask you how you are.

Of course, do not stop at greetings. Make sure that you also observe proper courtesy at all times. At the same time, make sure that you say "Thank you" or "You're welcome" when you do not have the opportunity yet to greet someone just yet. Even when you are not being heard by the entire room, people will still be able to observe that you are being nice to the people whom you are talking to. That will make you more approachable for the people that you want to build networks with.

5 Master the art of eye contact

Eye contact is an art, a pinnacle of non-verbal communication. Making good impressions are based not only on what you say and do, but also on how you convince people based on the way you say and do.

For instance, smiling may be a wonderful sight, but smiling without looking at the other person is a waste of time and effort. Smile, and show that you mean it by looking the other person in the eye in a pleasant, good-natured manner. This also applies to saying greetings and giving handshakes.

Maintaining an eye contact also promotes the idea that you are not only confident in expressing yourself, but that you are also interested on what another person is saying to you. Great eye contact also allows you to have connection with the other person who wants to meet your gaze. With eye contact alone, you can send a meaningful message to the person whom you want to make a connection with, even before you introduce yourself.

6 Dress appropriately

Dressing appropriately is rooted to knowing what occasion you are dressing for. Oftentimes, people are well aware of the dress code for a particular event but still stick to the belief that "no one will follow this dress code anyway". How many black tie parties have you attended with a couple of guests wearing dresses that are too short or even jeans?

Dressing according to the occasion means that you do not only prepare for the event, but that you also know what you are getting yourself into. It shows people that you have the right to be in the same event as them, and that you have something in common with them. Neglecting to show that to the people whom you want to connect with will automatically make them feel uneasy around you.

The purpose of dressing appropriately is not so much about blending in with the crowd, but about valuing the occasion and the hosts. Whether or not other attendees, participants, or guests will follow the dress code, you should be the better person and show that you adhered to what was advised. As the saying goes, "It is better to be overdressed than underdressed." When in doubt, go more formal than casual. For job interviews, meetings, and professional events, a pair of slacks or a skirt, a button-down shirt, and closed shoes are a no-fail outfit ensemble.

7 Be punctual

Being punctual is synonymous to showing respect. There's nothing worse than coming late and giving excuses that nobody wants to hear. Whether it's traffic or a simple lack of discernment and preparation, excuses are what make an unprofessional and unlikeable person.

That also means that a person who often shows up in an event late is a person who is not really keen on meeting people – a mark of a person who is only interested in himself. With that said, try to avoid making this impression especially if your motivation in going to any event is to market yourself and create networks. Not only do people have better things to do than wait for your arrival, you also miss a lot of opportunities when you arrive late. You will never know which important person has already left or had become too busy to entertain you when you come in during the middle of the gathering.

Showing up on time or even earlier means that you value the other person and his or her time. Remember that they also have some other place to go to after meeting with you, and have other tasks to do. Whether it is a party, a meeting, or a casual coffee sit-down with a new colleague, be responsible by being punctual.

8 Do your research

Doing your research is applicable when you are anticipating to meet someone, whether a potential employer, network, or colleague. This entails knowing about the person or people you will be meeting even before you meet them. Thanks to technology and the Internet, this is now possible.

If possible, make it a point to obtain the guest list of any possible networking event that you intend to attend. If you have a Facebook invitation, then take the time to check out who clicked on the Going button – doing so will give you an idea of the specific number of people who are going to the event and what these guests are like. If you want to check out their profiles, all you need to do is to hover over their names and click on their profile links. Doing so will not take much of your time, but will give you enormous advantage during the day of the event.

It doesn't hurt to Google their names or the company they work with. Check out their LinkedIn profile or Google+. This will help you gauge the interaction that you will have with them and maybe even give you something to talk about.

Why does reading about who you are going to meet matter nowadays? It is because the people whom you are expecting to meet probably think of doing the same thing as well. Because it is now possible for you to have an idea on what the people you are going to meet are like, there is no room for having no common ground anymore. You also have an idea on how to behave on a particular location or how to dress according to the occasion. That means that if you are still wondering how you can probably break the ice with people whom you are going to meet, or that you have doubts on whether they are going to like you during your initial meeting, you may need a little help from the Internet.

What should you research for? You definitely want to know what the other person is interested in. Take the time to read about his activities and what he does on his pastime. Also, remember to read about things that he probably does not like or have the slightest interest in so you know what you can avoid.

If possible, read about the line of work that the other person has. Read about his work experience and possible recognitions. If he has publications, then read them as well. That will allow you to have an idea on what this person is passionate about and how he will choose his words as a professional.

When researching about companies, try to unearth information that not a lot of people know. For instance, you can mention about a recognition or award that the company received, or an article promoting them online. This will show how interested you are, and will give more room for them to discuss with you. It will make you stand out, giving off a good impression.

9 Be remembered

When all has been said and done in your initial meeting and you feel like you've made a good and lasting impression, don't stop just yet.

Always make it a point that the other person will remember you. Busy people have loads of other people to meet within a day, and it is likely that your new network might forget you.

Prevent this by always carrying a bunch of business cards with you. It is a plus if your business card is smartly designed and unique, translating your great personality into a small piece of card. No matter how seemingly mundane, giving someone your business card amps up the chances of you being remembered by a hundred percent. Don't forget to politely ask for the other person's card as well.

When it is time to make an exit, make sure that you do not just leave – the point is to make sure that the people whom you just met will feel thankful that you have met. That will give you an assurance that the person whom you have introduced yourself to will remember you.

10 Re-connect

Once you meet someone, never let them go, at least metaphorically. After exchanging cards, you now have your foot in the door and the opportunities for re-connecting are endless.

Add the new people you've met on your professional online accounts such as LinkedIn, Google+, and your email list. You may want to think twice about adding them on social networking and sharing sites such as Facebook, Twitter, or Instagram, especially if your profiles share too much personal information. Remember, your networks are meant to be prospective employers, colleagues, and business partners. Save the casual online socializations for later.

You can also send them a simple text saying how it was a pleasure to meet them. If you want to go the professional route, sending an e-mail is most appropriate. You can add a few links to sites or resources that were part of your conversation, such as a link to an interesting article or a video of a talk you discussed about. This makes your e-mail more valuable and memorable.

Who knows, maybe the other person is looking forward to meeting you again? That's when you know you've made a good, lasting impression.

CHAPTER 3

LEARNING THE SECRETS OF RAPPORT

When it comes to building a network and including a person in your link, you need to understand that rapport is everything. Once you are able to establish rapport to the people that you are trying to connect to, you will see that even the people whom you just recently met are willing to cooperate with you and are more likely to respond positively to any invitation or request that you have for them.

What is Rapport?

Rapport is the relationship that you have with another person who allows you to make the other person feel that you are in harmony. As a result, the other person feels that it is easier for him to convey ideas when you are around. At the same time, other people will also feel that they understand you better.

Sometimes, rapport happens instantly with another person, especially if the two of you are the same in the first place. You may feel that you just "hit it off" during the first meeting, and that you have no problem trying to make him remember you or even agree to some of your propositions. When you meet someone whom you manage to just "hit it off" during an event, then you know that that person is for keeps.

Building rapport is natural – you will realize that rapport is nature's way of making living things coexist with each other in order for them to have access to the resources that they need. If you believe that you cannot exist without other people and that other people allow you to reach opportunities that you cannot attain on your own, then you understand what rapport can do to everyone who uses it in their daily lives.

Rapport is also the secret weapon of the most successful sales personnel – instead of forcing a person to buy his product, he instead sells his friendship to the person who he wants to convert into his client. By doing so, he becomes sure that this particular client will think of every way to help him and will continue his patronage, should he come knocking on his door again.

How to Build Rapport

Building rapport is natural for everyone. To build a harmonious relationship for another person, you just need to observe the following rules:

1. Make sure that the other person perceives you as someone who can help him. That means that he should not perceive you as a threat.

2. See to it that you find ways to relate to each other. Finding a mutual ground for your relationship to take off is a must.

3. Always assure the other person that you are someone who will be able to help him solve his problems. If the skill set that he needs is not within your reach, then you can find someone else who can help him.

When you think about it, building rapport is simply thinking that you need to care for the person that you are trying to build a relationship with. When you communicate to other people that you do care for their best interests, you will be able to minimize conflict and establish that you will be getting mutual benefit once you enter an amicable relationship.

CHAPTER 4

KEYS 11-20: BECOME A GREAT CONVERSATIONALIST

Now that you've made a good, lasting impression and have gained new networks, the next step is to sustain this relationship. It is possible that you have made a positive initial impression, only for the other person to learn that you may not be as great as they first thought you were.

Of course, everyone has their own manifestations of greatness as well as areas of improvement. In your case, be the person that will be remembered and be liked, to the point that your networks jump to the opportunity of meeting you again.

Make that Impression your Commitment

How do you become likeable, trusted, and influential, anyway? The secret is in being the best communicator and conversationalist. After all, we communicate and converse on a daily basis. Often, we rely on what we say and how we say it, forgetting what the other person is saying and how he or she is saying it as well.

The way you carry a conversation serves as your follow-up to that firm handshake or that welcoming smile that you flashed when you saw a person come in the room. Conversations show your depth of character, as well as your background as a person. The way you talk to a person will also show how genuine that interest that you showed him is when you introduced yourself to him.

Redeem Yourself during the Conversation

If you feel that you have made a lousy introduction of yourself, then carrying a meaningful conversation is the second chance that you get to make the person want to network with you. This means that if you think you have made a weak entrance or that you have made a blunder during your first meeting, then take the opportunity to be remembered as a great contact the moment you have the chance to speak.

While it is difficult to change what you have created as your first impression, people are quick to forgive a good conversationalist. Good conversationalists are full of fun and intelligence, with their charms often lying within their words. Most people accept this as the truth, which allows them to consider the conversation as part of another person's introduction.

Starting a Conversation

If you are the type who is daunted about having to make the first move, then do not be afraid, even if you are in a crowded room filled with people who have already made friends with others. If you want to start networking in an event and you can't find a good starting point, then the best person to talk to first is the one who is not talking to anyone.

Why that person, instead of the host, or the CEO whom you have been trying to get into your contact list? The reason is simple – everybody else is still busy trying to create their own network, and are probably engaging a group. In order for you to weave your way into a conversation, you need to test your communication skills first. The best way to do that is to talk to a person who seems to be distant from the rest of the crowd.

That person is most likely to be someone who has the same level of anxiety as yours – he may be a person who does not know anyone in the room and is waiting for every opportunity to leave the event, but cannot. Talking to that person means assuring him that it is alright for him to be in the event, and that it is okay for him to also network like the others. That will also make him feel that someone has genuine interest in him.

If you manage to hit it off with that person, you can encourage him to go with you as you introduce yourself to others. That would not only reduce your anxiety, but also enable yourself to ease in on group conversations.

What Should the Subject be About?

At this point, you should keep in mind that when it comes to conversations, whether striking a conversation or keeping one going, you need to understand that people are interested in themselves. That truth does not mean that it is a bad thing – people are simply focused on themselves and it is a human need to feel important. Once they feel that the stranger that they are talking to is interested in them and will do what it takes to make them feel valuable, they are more inclined to return the favor.

Of course, handling a conversation means that you also focus on how you appear to be talking to others. While most people think that talking to another person involves mere words, it is not – a great conversation is a mix of gestures, expressions, tone of voice, and subliminal body language. Words only come as secondary in importance.

In becoming a great conversationalist, the focus is not so much about you and the content of what you say that will sweep others off their feet; the spotlight is on the other person and how you can lead the conversation to make it a two-way exchange.

What good are flowery words and astounding content, when you have no clue how to deliver them the proper way? Here are networking keys 11-20, skills that you can carry with you and apply in every conversation you engage in.

11 Give affirmations

Affirmations are everything. To affirm means to encourage, and it also means that you find something pleasant or good in the person whom you are speaking to. More than merely expressing appreciation, affirmations also tell that there is something in the conversation that you both agree to. Like in most relationships, expressing this agreement promotes the idea that you both have a common ground, and that common ground prompts both of you to commit to each other, either by way of friendship or business.

This practice involves more than just giving an overflow of praise and compliments, but centering on another person's strengths and positive characteristics without sounding artificial. Often, people blurt out the first compliment they can think of, such as "I love your hair" or "Nice shoes". Although there's nothing wrong with these statements, a better way to affirm is to acknowledge the qualities that make a person unique and special. Examples of this include telling a person how you appreciate his or her humility, or generously talking about a recent achievement that this person has accomplished.

12 Mirror

Mirroring is a conversational skill that can serve not only to make the other person feel understood and heard, but also helps build trust and likeability on your part. This skill is similar to looking in the mirror but in the context of communication, wherein you reflect back to the person what he or she is saying.

Mirroring, in psychology, also means pacing. That means that by reflecting words or gestures of the person you are talking to, you are sending a message that both of you are in sync, and you are in the same page in the conversation. The idea that you both are doing the same thing also sends a powerful idea that you are the same in other aspects of life, and you are more likely to agree in other topics as well.

A good way to do this technique is to summarize what the other person is saying, in a way that shows that you fully understood him or her. Another effective mirroring technique is to somehow reflect the communication patterns of the person, such as tone of voice, speed of talking, and gestures. You can also mirror how another person dresses, and you may also observe that people who are wearing a similar attire are more likely to be at ease with each other, compared to those who are dressed differently. This is the secret that will guarantee likeable responses from the person you're communicating with, and will also allow you to communicate more ideas and network more effectively.

Such technique is not meant to manipulate people or mock them, but intended to make yourself be at the same pace and level as the person you are speaking with. For instance, if the person is conversing in a reserved, relaxed voice, it is very likely that he or she will respond better to someone who mirrors this pace, instead of someone who talks in a loud, hurried manner.

Mirroring is so powerful because its effect happens on a subconscious level. It is even possible for a person to realize that there is someone whom he is in sync with even from across the room! Once that person realizes that there is a person who is similar to him, he is more likely to be more approachable or even initiate contact.

13 Learn nonverbal and verbal cues

Mirroring and communicating entail knowing how to read and respond to non-verbal cues. Non-verbal communication is so influential that it determines the outcomes of a particular conversation. In fact, people communicate non-verbally without knowing it. Having the awareness and knowledge in reading non-verbal cues will definitely give you an edge when it comes to communicating with your networks.

While you are at it, also observe the words that the other person uses. For example, you may notice that a person may be using words such as "I see your point" or "I hear you" whenever he expresses agreement with you. These words that refer to their senses hold a lot of clues on how you can effectively communicate with them. You may notice that people are actually more receptive to you if you mirror their verbal cues.

14 Ask the right questions

The questions you ask determine your intelligence and ability to listen. People who ask the right questions are perceived as curious and genuinely interested in what the other person is saying.

Asking the right questions will also allow you to make the right clarifications at the right time, especially if you are truly at a loss in a conversation. Take note that some people avoid having to ask questions and simply agree with everything that is being thrown in the conversation – avoid this mistake, since agreeing to something that you do not understand may lead into awkward encounters in the future or missing out on what a person is really great at.

To be able to ask the right questions, you need to be able to listen intently. Whether or not you understand what was said, there is always room for questions. Try asking more open-ended queries (questions that can be answered with more than a yes or no) to keep the conversation flowing.

Of course, keep in mind that asking the right questions should be balanced with revealing information about yourself. Asking questions for most parts of the conversation will make the other person think that you are being a busybody, if not nosey. On the other hand, revealing information about yourself too often in the conversation will make them feel that you are bound to overshare. When it comes to making a perfect conversation, the balance is in the mix.

15 Make it about the other person, not just about you

In relation to asking the right questions, the conversation should never be one-way. This means that it should be an exchange of words, ideas, statements, questions; a sharing instead of a monologue. Unless a particular conversation is meant to give instructions or a lecture, you should not polarize the conversation in any way. To make it about the other person and not just your own, always ask follow-up questions to stories and ideas then state your side or your opinion. After that, always ask the other person, "What do you think about that?"

16 Bridge cultural differences effectively

Cultural differences come in all forms. These are not exclusive to relations with people of different race or nationalities, but those of different beliefs, upbringing, personalities, and so on. In short, we all experience cultural differences on a regular basis. To some extent, we are all culturally different. The mere fact that we come from different family backgrounds, demeanor, and locations already makes every interaction a melting pot of cultural variety.

However, it is important to realize that people who belong to the same cultural traditions or sensitivities are more likely to bond together or belong to the same network. You can think of it as similar to the idea that people who mirror each other will possibly link together or desire to belong group – it is just that people who hail from the same traditions are bonded as if they come from the same family. They are also more likely to shun people who do not observe the same traditions or have an opposing belief.

For this reason, it is crucial to remember that the key to bridging cultural differences is sensitivity. There is nothing worse than being careless about what you say or do, with no regard for other people's sensibilities. To avoid this, it is always best to ask. Better yet, try getting information about your networks, such as details of their place of origin, the languages they speak, religion, among others. This will help you gauge what words or behaviors to avoid.

The good news is that there is always room for understanding. After all, nobody shouldn't box anybody up and stereotype a particular group of people just because of their background. Always remember to be open and sensitive, and you will be able to carry a conversation with someone who is culturally different from you.

17 Acknowledge feelings

Acknowledging feelings is actually pretty simple yet it requires a great deal of openness and humility. People tend to mask and suppress their feelings and get on with their lives everyday. The truth is, bottling up your feelings is dangerous. You might end up shattering that bottle of emotions and spewing ugly words from your mouth without warning.

Acknowledging another person's feelings or beliefs goes a long way. It makes it possible for another person that while you may have a differing opinion, you make him understand that you understand that you can agree that you disagree. That makes the other person feel that he is free to express his emotions and ideas without feeling that he is going to be met with opposition. That also welcomes the idea in the conversation that once thoughts are communicated well, you may arrive at a common ground once again.

By creating this atmosphere whenever there is a debate within a conversation, you will be able to guarantee the people whom you are trying to build a network with that you are still on their side, and the difference that you both may be expressing is essential in making everyone realize that you are being diplomatic and you are trying to bridge differences for a more dynamic relationship.

A healthy way to communicate feelings is to say it as it is without judging the other person. Instead of saying "you", say "I', also known as an "I- Statement". It is always best to own up to what you think and feel, instead of projecting it to the other person.

Should you need to voice out that you disagree with the opinion of others, see to it that you state your reason first. This will create the idea that you have carefully thought of your reasons before stating that you disagree with another person's opinion right off the bat. By stating why you are disagreeing with someone's opinion first, you are encouraging a healthy debate fueled by rationality, instead of clashes of emotions that will not have any resolve.

18 Have empathy

Empathy is a powerful tool that you can apply in any interaction or conversation. Empathy can be summarized as the ability to place oneself in another person's shoes and understand where he or she is coming from. Of course, it is impossible to understand someone 100%. Part of having empathy is accepting that even if you cannot fully understand someone, you are committed to being kind and considerate.

Empathizing with someone also allows the other person to know that you are capable of accepting the flaws of another person, without making mistakes affect your intention of including him in your life. That allows him to regroup and start over in his place in the conversation, and continue sharing with the rest of the group.

19 Accept compliments

When someone compliments you, what is your usual response? Do you brush off the compliment and say, "Oh, stop it" in a bashful way, or do you divert it to the other person and say, "No, you're prettier!" If you do, you may need to rethink that action. By accepting praise, you are acknowledging that the idea that the impression that you have made on another person is true. That creates a favorable atmosphere to proceed to a conversation.

The best way to handle praise is to freely accept it without sounding too proud. Saying a simple "Thank you" is enough, but you can add up to it by saying something that also compliments the other person, such as "I can say the same thing about you as well." Openly accepting compliments modestly gives off a great attitude without sounding vain.

20 Offer something valuable

Lastly, don't forget that every interaction and conversation is an opportunity to show your worth and offer something valuable. You never know if the person you're conversing with in a party could be your future boss or business partner.

Offering something valuable can be done in different ways. Try to sneak in some trivia or unique information that is applicable to the conversation, or share book titles and authors that you think the other person can benefit from. You can also send links to resources, such as relevant videos and articles. As for advice giving, it is best to leave it for those who are directly asking for it. Don't give advice off-hand because not everyone might be open to it. Offering something valuable means handing something that the person would want to receive, not something that would offend or irritate.

Being a great conversationalist requires some practice, but with time and effort, you will get there.

CHAPTER 5

DEALING WITH SHYNESS OR SOCIAL ANXIETY

Since the previous chapter covered starting and handling meaningful conversations, you may be wondering how useful those key tips are if you are the type who feels uncomfortable around other people. If you are daunted about having to speak to people that you barely know, do not feel discouraged to network. Believe it or not, there are a lot of people who managed to build an extensive network of contacts, despite having to struggle with shyness or social anxiety.

The Truth about Shyness

You may realize that networking makes it imperative for a person to be confident, but what should one do if he really lacks self-esteem? Would that be the end of the opportunity to meet other people? Of course not. The truth is that 75% of the population deals with a degree of social anxiety. Another fact is that glossophobia, or the fear of public speaking, remains to be the most widespread fear in America. When you think about it, there are more people who are afraid to talk to people in a public place than those who are afraid of dying.

The lack of self-esteem is natural for everyone. Nervousness happens when you are about to do something that you are unsure of. While your career will depend on how you network at a great degree, you do not need to worry about how you are going to make impressions or go around talking to people if you are anxious. Before going out there and making a connection, it is best for you to understand why you feel afraid when you are about to engage people whom you do not know.

Anxiety arises when your body prepares for something that you do not sure what the outcome is. You feel nervous for something that you are unprepared for, and that is something that you will regularly feel if you do not make the right preparations for a networking event. For that reason, it is imperative for you to do your research about the guests that you are going to meet and come to gatherings on time in order for you to cope with the situation. Not only would doing so make you appear professional, you would also be able to buy the time and prepare yourself before you approach someone. You will also be able to predict if someone is going to talk to you during a gathering, and then get used to the feeling of talking.

People are as Nervous as You Are

One of the things that shy and anxious people do when they are daunted by the presence of others is to focus on themselves. They become so conscious about their actions to the point that they forget the other person. The result is very predictable – they lose eye contact, they become increasingly awkward, and then they lose focus on the topic of the conversation. The next thing that may happen is that they will give a rather weak excuse to get themselves out of the situation. When that happens, you may be losing the opportunity to learn something from the possible contact that you just have met.

You can avoid all these by keeping this thought in your mind – relax, the people around you are focusing on themselves and may have the same thoughts as you. You do not have to focus on becoming comfortable around other people in a networking event. If you focus your attention on them, instead of yourself, then you will automatically switch your line of thinking. Because you would realize that they are also nervous to be there, you will be more concerned on how you can make them feel comfortable.

At this point, you will see that the more you observe people in meet ups or gatherings, the more you will observe that most people are actually consciously watching themselves if they are going to have a slip in their introductions or conversations. They do not even notice how nervous you are! The reason is that they are all trying to avoid mistakes.

Make People Comfortable Around You

How important is it that you make people you do not know comfortable? The reason is this: the calmer you are, the more effective you become in holding a conversation. Of course, it is impossible to be calm when the people who are trying to talk to you are full of jitters themselves.

If you are aware that you cannot maintain your composure, focus on the other person and see if he is probably as nervous as you are – see if he is making blunders with his words, or if there are beads of sweat forming in his forehead. When you observe that they are exhibiting signs of anxiety but are trying their best to converse with you, offer them a drink or a seat. Once they eased up, tell them that you are actually nervous to be in that event, but you would not pass up the opportunity to be with amazing people.

Admitting to the fact that you are nervous will not only make these people feel relieved that they are not alone in their dilemma, but also make them feel that they have something in common with you. Now, you have established a common ground for you to talk about!

Once you feel confident about speaking to these people, you can find a way to speak to the other guests as well. Of course, do not forget to ask for their calling cards and give them yours, too.

CHAPTER 6

KEYS 21-30: LEARN "NETIQUETTE"

The advent of technology has allowed people to communicate in a multitude of ways, one of which is through online tools and platforms. Online communication channels are endless, especially when it comes to networking, socializing, and sharing.

You Will Meet a Lot of People Online

With that said, you need to keep in mind that the personality that you have online will make a great impact on how people will see you when you meet in person. Because people do not see the nuances of your gestures or facial expressions, which may greatly explain why you behave or soften some of the words that you may use, you need to exercise caution whenever you post photos or say something online.

While most people may not treat social media or online presence seriously, there are a lot of people who matter to you who do. Most of them are those in your network who will desire to conduct a background check, such as employers, business partners, or clients. The reason is simple – they want to know if the identity that you have online matches the personality that you show them whenever you see each other in person.

You also need to remember that people do rely on technology nowadays to have a deeper understanding of a person they barely know. For example, a person that you have recently made an acquaintance may want to know what kind of books you read or what university you went to. He may also want to have some feedback about the work that you have done. All these information are easily accessible online. When you think about it, all the people who you meet will also have an idea about what you do on a regular day when you are out to enjoy personal time, or when you are meeting people on your other networks. The information that they may get online may or may not conflict their impression of you, and that would affect the relationship that you are trying to build.

Keep Your Online Image Sanitized

While people may express the idea that people should accept whatever they post on their personal space, it is also very important that while your accounts can only be touched by you, whatever you say on the Web creates the idea that people can comment on it or even share it. Because networking is still based on word of mouth and recommendations, it is best to keep an online profile that makes people compelled to invite others to connect with you. Of course, you want people to recommend you to others the way you want them to, and for that reason, provide your network a reference that you would want them to do. That's right, your LinkedIn and Facebook account will be their reference, so make sure that those spaces will give you positive results.

In this day and age, your online identity and presence are extremely important in maintaining your networks and building relationships. One vital skill that you need is netiquette, the etiquette required in online interactions. It is not enough to be polite in actual interactions; you should also practice good manners and sound conduct online.

Here are keys 21 to 30, most of which have been derived from The Core Rules of Netiquette by Virginia Shea.

21 Interact the way you would offline

The ultimate key to practicing netiquette is treating an online exchange as parallel to personal, face-to-face, offline interactions. Virginia Shea refers to this as recognizing the human. After all, we are still primarily interacting with people, not robots.

Common courtesy practices, such as greetings and proper addressing are still very much needed in online interactions. Typing in all capital letters should be avoided unless necessary in the online conversation, as this might be interpreted as shouting. Use proper punctuations and end the online conversation politely.

22 Know your cyber place

Cyberspace wasn't created equal. Some sites are more formal while others are casual. Know your place in cyberspace.

Treat online spaces like you are attending an event – you would realize that while some forums or Facebook groups feel like you are in a seminar, there are those spaces that will make you realize that you are in a college party. If you are able to successfully identify the kind of space you are in, then you will be able to match that space with an appropriate behavior. If possible, it would also be wise to change your online avatar or profile image to better suit the space that you want to interact others with.

For instance, if you are participating in an online forum about a particular interest such as celebrity news, it is perfectly fine to go all out on emoticons, shortcuts such as LOL (laughing out loud) and ROFL (rolling on the floor laughing), and casual chatter. However, if you are part of something academic or professional such as an online class or a TED talk, you might want to be more discerning of how you interact online.

23 Be considerate of others' time and bandwidth

Being considerate of others is not exclusive to offline interactions. In fact, being online means exerting more effort to respect others and their resources, in this case their time and bandwidth.

Most people who interact online would want others to be considerate when it comes to taking turns on a group chat, or sharing documents and photos. While some consider the Internet to be a space of abundance, making music, videos, and photos to be considered as shareable content, there are those who would want to stick to reading texts instead. For that reason, it pays to share the content that other people would want to view.

Oversharing may seem like your initial impulse, but do you think your online contacts are equally interested in everything you want to share? You might be eating up their time and bandwidth without you realizing it.

24 Write good content

The last thing you want is for someone to Google your name, only to be greeted by search results of your negative and rash online interactions. As much as possible, always write content in a positive, constructive manner.

Content is the king online, and without good content, you will never be able to compel people to network with you. For that reason, it is important that you update information about you as often as you can. That means that if you are determined to have strong online presence, make sure that you delete your old blogs and maintain your recent ones. Also, make sure that something new and relevant is found on your social media accounts. That does not only tell people more about your interests, but also say that you have the time to inform people new things about your areas of expertise.

However, you will only be able to influence people if you are stating your knowledge and your opinions in a positive and welcoming manner. Should your aim is to start a debate, make sure that you are encouraging people to have a fair and friendly argument, which would be enriching for everyone in the end.

Stating your personal opinion online is one thing, but doing so in a hostile way is not attractive to your networks and colleagues, or to anyone for that matter. Be on your toes at all times when it comes to writing online, as these can be easily documented, saved, and unearthed with just a few clicks.

25 Share what you know

The Internet is the best place to share and extract information. According to Virginia Shea, the strength of the Net is in its numbers. Practices like crowdsourcing are becoming very popular, wherein online users gather others' opinions, ideas, recommendations, and even funds.

Your generosity may just be your ticket to a new network or community. Offering something valuable doesn't have to be in the form of money; you can share your knowledge and expertise as well. There are many ways to be generous in the online world— share what you have and what you know in online forums, crowdsourcing websites, social networking sites, and resource sites such as Scribd and Amazon.

If you find someone in your network who is also sharing relevant information about your fields of interest, or you find a work that you like, make sure that you also share their content. That does not only allow you to engage with the person and improve your relationship online, but also puts in the special effort to make your contacts get introduced to his work.

26 Be the light, not the flame

In the Core Rules of Netiquette, Virginia Shea addresses "flaming". This pertains to the outright expression of intense emotions and ideas, an inevitable occurrence in the online world.

A common example of flaming is a heated debate in the comments section of a YouTube video. Although you may have equally strong opinions about a particular topic or issue, try holding your tongue as much as possible (or your fingers from impulsively typing on your keyboard). Of course, you have the right to express what you think and feel, but you can do so in a constructive manner.

Instead of feeding the flame and adding to the intensity of the argument, be the light. This means trying to balance out the discussion by acknowledging the sides of each party, stating your own viewpoint, and recognizing that flaming will achieve nothing. Be an online peacemaker and mediator.

27 Give value to privacy

Privacy is a sensitive yet necessary subject in the online world. Some online users are careful with their privacy and even anonymity, while others are a bit lax. When it comes to this aspect, it is best to be more private than be too visible online.

You respect a person's privacy by ensuring that you do not share or link information that another person may feel offensive or damaging to his reputation. At the same time, you should also feel that it is your responsibility to report offensive posts regarding people in your network and inform them that such posts exist in order for them to review their privacy policies.

Respecting others' privacy preference is imperative. As for your own, there are ways to edit and re-set your privacy settings on your online accounts. Be knowledgeable about them and stay safe and secure. Valuing your privacy also helps filter information and keeps your online presence as pristine as possible.

28 Respect differences

In the online world, it is very likely that you will interact with people from different backgrounds. The beauty of the Internet lies in the user's capacity to connect with people across the globe with a few clicks.

Part of netiquette involves being mindful of differences and cultural diversities. Be sure to stay away from offensive, racist, sexist, and insulting online behavior. The goal is to promote inclusivity and harmony, not divide and disrespect.

For this reason, make sure that you do not only post cultural and religious-sensitive information, but also curate posts that you allow others to share with you. Letting people know that you shun opinions that may be offending from your social media platforms also encourage positive behavior on your network. Doing so goes a long way – people will learn that you are only interested in engaging with them when they have helpful posts, but that you are also willing to champion the online rights of others.

29 Be kind

Kindness is slowly being taken for granted online. At the end of the day, your offline and online interactions reflect who you are as a person. Being unkind can leave a mark, literally, as online information can be stored, saved, screenshot, and shared.

Of course, you are not just motivated to practice kindness out of fear and requirement, but out of sincerity and authenticity. Being kind can go a long way in helping you keep your networks and build relationships.

30 Regularly clean up and update your profile

Your online footprints will be there forever. You never know when a network or colleague is digging up your online involvements and getting to know you through your online profiles.

For instance, employers looking to hire new people are often on the lookout on websites such as LinkedIn and job search platforms. Social networking sites are also a great place to discover information about a prospective new employee.

Make it a habit to clean up and update your online profiles, especially those that are set to public. You never know when a potential employer or partner is going through your profile and weighing if they want to reconnect or contact you.

Important Note: Maintain a Clean Online Image at All Costs

If you are trying to build a successful network online, see to it that your online record is truly clean. Run a check of your name or your images online to check for uploads or webpages that may discredit you. If you have blogs or spare Facebook accounts that contain rants about a previous workplace or anything that would lead people into thinking that you lack professionalism, delete them. You can also ask for the assistance from the site's webmaster to delete any unwanted posts that may get linked back to you.

Why does this step matter? The reason is that there are people who can go over and beyond when it comes to researching your background, without meaning any harm. However, accidentally stumbling into these "skeletons" may dissuade them from connecting with you, or make you want to offer an unneeded explanation for things that already belong to the past. To prevent that unnecessary and preventable problem, make sure that your online reputation is spotless.

CHAPTER 7

KEYS 31-40: MAINTAIN NETWORKS

In the previous chapters, you learned how to make a good and lasting impression, be a great conversationalist, and practice netiquette. The next step is to know how to maintain your networks. Getting people to like and trust you is not enough; you have to make a considerable amount of effort to sustain these new relationships and contacts.

Remind People About You

When you create networks, you only have one thing in mind – to establish yourself as a go-to person whenever your expertise is needed. At the same time, you also need to make them realize that you know someone whom they probably need in any case they do need someone else.

How do you do that? You need to make sure that you are constantly engaging with each member of your network, no matter who they are. You need to establish that despite their different backgrounds or fields of interest, you always have something to offer them. This creates the reciprocity that you need to get from any network, which is an exchange of services and building each other up by providing each other's needs.

Maintaining Network is Harder than Creating One

People value consistency, and when you are on the road to expanding your reach and establishing yourself in your field, you may find that staying in touch with everyone is tougher than going out to meet people. However, being able to maintain your network is the first step to make sure that the people who you know would want to stay connected to you.

Some people make the mistake of asking for favors from those whom they just met – you may probably not think of doing that, but there are twists and turns in life that may prompt you to do that. However, how would these people want to help you? You begin by continuing your interest in them and extending your help first. This way, you can create an added value for yourself, which is that you are the dependable part of their network, who is capable of going out of your way in order to offer your assistance.

Of course, that does not stop there. Since you would want to keep your network for a very long time, you need to keep on engaging with people, even those whom you are not likely to work with soon. By keeping in touch with them, you are able to establish a relationship with them, even when they know that they cannot help you yet. What you are creating when you do this is more mutual grounds for both of you, which would allow you to discover latent interests, or better yet, skills that you can harness for mutual benefit.

Keys 31-40 will teach you how to effectively keep and even develop your relationships with your colleagues.

31 Utilize social media

In Chapter 3, you learned about netiquette and how important it is to be well mannered and considerate online. With this knowledge, you should be able to utilize social media effectively.

Maximize the features of social media by keeping up to date with your colleagues. For instance, always make sure to greet them on special occasions such as birthdays and anniversaries. Congratulate them on their achievements and engage with them whenever they are expressing an opinion on a topic that is very important to them.

Since social media makes it possible for you to use the Like or Share options, you will also be able to tell people on your network that you have been following their posts and you are still open to conversations, even when you are not together. Such gestures are always welcome and appreciated.

32 Don't bombard them with emails

E-mailing is highly effective and dependable when it comes to maintaining your networks. However, be sensitive enough not to bombard your contacts with daily e-mails that will just flood their inbox. Try to be discerning and only share relevant information. The last thing you want is your e-mail to be dumped in the spam folder or worse, be deleted entirely.

Keep in mind that you only want to engage with people whom you are sharing things that you need to enrich your life or to give you an advantage in your career. You do not want to receive news that you do not care about or would not make a difference, and for that reason, make sure that you extend the courtesy of not pushing details about yourself and your interests to people that may not really care for them. Make sure that you only extend information that will make them want to engage with you, and not something that may lead you into being branded as a spammer or a hard seller.

33 Group your networks

Grouping your networks entails sorting them into different categories, whether on your mailing list, Facebook account, or an online group. This will help you reconnect with them better, send relevant messages, and even remember them altogether.

It would also help to keep a list of people whom you desire to connect with more often, either because they will give you better opportunities or that you are inspired by them. You will realize that by grouping people and creating a contact list, you will be able to remember those in your network better. That eliminates the danger of addressing someone differently or making errors in your conversations or referrals.

34 Tailor your messages

In relation to grouping your networks, make it a habit to tailor and customize your messages. It is easy to send a group message to a particular network group, but try going the extra mile and make your messages more personal and heartfelt.

Remember that the sweetest word for any person is his own name, so make sure that you address everyone in your network with their names every chance that you get. That also gives the impression that you are the type of person who can remember every detail of conversations that you have had, and that you are reaching out to continue those conversations.

35 Offer help

Offering help is an excellent way to maintain your networks. If a colleague is in need of any help, whether it be new information, a need for specific resources such as books, or simple manual help, try to be participative and volunteer to offer help in whatever way you can.

By telling people that you are willing to help them, with or without anything in return, you are also saying that you are an expert in your field of interest. You are also saying that it does not take a lot of effort whenever you assist someone. That does not only encourage other people to extend their help whenever you need it, it also tells people that you are genuinely interested in the success of others. If you are not able to extend any assistance that they would need, they would still remember that you are interested in helping and would keep that in mind.

36 Refer

If you are unable to offer help, refer people who can. Giving referrals are not only perfect for helping your networks, but also helping the people you refer to make new networks themselves. This will expand your web of networks and may even help build a community. There's nothing more fulfilling than creating a community of people that work for a common purpose.

When you refer other people to help out, you are not making the impression that you are not willing to get the job done, especially if you are more than capable of handling the task. By referring people, you acknowledge that there are those who can be better than you or deserve the opportunity better. That does not only indicate that you have people in your contact list that can be readily utilized for the benefit of others, but you also display humility and mindfulness to the needs of others.

Keep in mind that there is no shame in telling people that there is someone out there who is better than you – that saves you from extending a half-hearted support to people in your network, when you know that the job could have been done better. When you want to keep people in your network, always think that you always want the best for them.

Referring others for a project also makes people in your network realize that you do care for other's expertise and that you are willing to do what it takes to promote their skills or give them a chance to showcase their talent. It also allows you to expand your network by being known as a person that share opportunities with the people that you know. Because of this, other people would also be encouraged to do the same favor for you and the people that you know. When that happens, people would want to stay connected with you because they become aware that being within your network means more options for their growth.

37 Invite

Building relationships and maintaining networks involves having common interests. If you know any event, seminar, or occasion that you think can be of help to your networks and colleagues do not hesitate to invite them. There's a great chance that you can help add up to their growth and professional development, inevitably strengthening your relationship with them.

Inviting other people to attend does not only allow you to express that you want them to be a part of your project or that you can go with someone to a function, it also tells them that you are willing to share your resources to your colleagues and peers. While that does strengthen your relationship, you are also encouraging them to share their own resources for your benefit. What is more compelling to want another person to grow than knowing that you would also be with that person to the top? When you allow the people in your network to know that you would continually include them in your plans and functions, they would want to become more valuable to you and offer additional support. Not only are you prompting them to be more visible, you are also encouraging them to grow.

38 Keep your word

Nobody likes a wishy-washy person who does not know how to keep promises. If you commit to something, do it. Keeping your word builds trust and enhances your reputation.

Perhaps there is nothing relationship-tarnishing than not being able to do something despite of a promise. When you immediately beg off from a commitment that you have previously made, you are making the impression that the other plans that you have in mind are definitely more important than the person that you made a promise to. That also creates the impression that you can be fickle-minded and that you do not know how to lock your schedules to accommodate requests or invitations. This does not only hurt the people in your network every time you make a last-minute rejection, but also make them think that they cannot trust you to do well when they offer you bigger opportunities.

Constantly breaking your word can escalate, and that would definitely hurt your reputation in no time at all. Not only would people not want to refer you because of the fear that you would bring them down, they would also want to kick you out of their own network and grant opportunities that were initially for you to someone else.

39 Participate in professional groups

Professional groups that are aligned to your interests or field are always worth your time. You can either join a group that meets up regularly, or take part in an online community. Join groups where your networks are active to further maintain your connection and relationship with them.

40 Meet up

If your time permits, try to meet up with networks that you consider as close contacts, or ones whom you want to get to know better. A simple get-together over coffee will suffice, or try doing something together, such as attending a workshop or listening to a lecture about a topic you are equally interested in. Nothing beats the power of physical, face-to-face interaction in maintaining and cultivating relationships.

While there is a way for you to converse with people online, meeting up with people over drinks or a meal tells them that you are willing to clear up your schedule in order to give them the time of the day when you can assist them with their needs or catch up with their lives. That immediately strengthens the bond that you have with a person. Take note that you do not have to just meet people to do something professional – you are not requiring them to go see you because you want to do work. By doing activities like having a brunch together or playing a round of golf, you are insinuating that you also know have to have fun, and you want people that you are in touch with to have fun with you.

A Note on Who You Should Constantly Communicate With

You may be thinking that maintaining contact with everyone in your network is tough, especially if there are hundreds of people in your contact list. Attempting to spend time with everyone in your network is a sure way to spread yourself thin – a networking error that would prompt you to become less effective when it comes to offering assistance or keeping your word.

Most people do try to keep in touch with everyone that they know on a regular basis, even when they know that it is simply impossible to do so. Think about this: how many people in your network really does matter to you? Who are the people that you truly want to engage with, and who are the ones that genuinely interest you? Surely, not all of them. For that reason, it is very important that you identify the people that should get majority of your time and dedicate your resources into developing your relationship with them.

At this point, keep a mental list of the people whom you genuinely like and will help enrich your life as a professional or will take the time to build your skills. There are not a lot of them, so it should be easy for you to identify all of them. Now, keep in mind that these people in your list are the ones who will make you feel glad that you are assisting them, because they automatically make you feel valuable. They are also the ones who instantly gratify your needs and who are willing to exert the same amount of effort that you have given them.

CHAPTER 8

KEY 41: CONSTANTLY LEARN AND IMPROVE

You are well on your way to career growth as you make good and lasting impressions, converse and communicate well, keep a positive online presence, and maintain your networks effectively.

Amid all these, you should never stop working on yourself. After all, you are your own marketer, manager, and advertiser. More than the words that you say, the impression that you make, or the content that you share online, your work and your personality will always speak for themselves. After all, cultivating and maintaining networks and relationships are all about creating more opportunities and promoting growth.

The biggest investment that you can make is on yourself— adding up to your knowledge, skills, and great attitude. Nobody can take these away from you. Having a knowledgeable mind, an extensive set of skills, and a developed attitude and persona are your best tools in networking and being the most likeable and sought-after person in your field.

To develop yourself, make it a point to attend seminars, workshops, and lectures that can help contribute more knowledge and skills in your chosen field. If money is an issue, there are so many free online courses that you can sign up for on the internet that you can take on your own time and pace, in the comforts of your home.

Encourage Learning Together

There are a lot of people in your network who share the same interests with you, and will probably have the resources that you need in order to expand your knowledge. Make the most out of your existing connections by asking for some resource materials or inviting them out and asking if they can teach you a thing or two over coffee.

By encouraging mentorship in your network, you do not only make people in your circle feel valuable because of their knowledge, but you also help them make a footprint that they are experts in their fields. It will also help to introduce them to people who are looking for the same information and will use their help. The people whom you seek assistance from will gladly open up their time to accommodate your request.

You will also be able to brush up on your existing tools of trade if you teach other members of your network and share what you know to the entire group. When you are teaching someone, you will realize that there are some details in your craft that you have already forgotten about, or that you would have rekindled interest in some fields that you did not really pay attention to. Not only would you have the motivation to study more, you would also be able to update your skills and have another set of expertise in no time at all.

Invest in Workshops and the Academe

If you still have more time in your hands, attend workshops or pursue another degree from a university. That would not only allow you to achieve higher education in a field that you are interested in, but also improve your academic record. Make sure that you include the new diploma or certificate in your résumé – that would make more people interested in networking with you, thanks to your additional academic achievement.

Read More

Constantly learning and improving also means investing on resource materials such as books, CDs, and other helpful references. You have the option to buy, borrow, or ask friends for copies or files. Try to set a goal when it comes to reading books; say, 10 books a year. That's 10 sources of knowledge already, 10 unique perspectives. Reading expands the mind and opens up your worldview, allowing you to have more understanding and empathy for people from all walks of life.

It also helps to know that CEOs and other people who are determined to expand their professional networks are those who actually spend time to read at least 5 books in a month. That means that there is no real excuse when it comes to expanding your knowledge. The more you read, the easier it becomes for you to find information that would help your network and also allow you to connect with people who are in other fields of interest.

Learning and improving yourself doesn't have to be academic or formal in approach. If you're not much of a reader or a seminar attendee, you can still develop and improve by associating yourself with wise, knowledgeable people. Often, these are persons who are much older than you. Whether it is a former professor, an expert in a particular field, or your elderly neighbor, you can always learn something from people who've had much more life experience than you.

Be a lifelong learner. Never stop developing yourself in whatever way you can. Learn a new language. Try a new hobby. This will increase your market value a hundred fold, making you even more wonderful, admired, and sought-after than you already are.

CHAPTER 9

THE MOST IMPORTANT KEY- KEY 42: BE AUTHENTIC

Finally, you have come to the final key in this book, key 42. You have read all about the different keys to building relationships, enhancing your networks, and creating influence. You may be asking— what is the ultimate key to being likeable and admired?

The answer is simple— be authentic.

It is Okay to Be Yourself

One of the major reasons why people suddenly experience having to burn bridges with those whom they previously connected with is because they are not the ones whom they are trying to promote. Some people have to feign that they belong to the top 1% when in fact, they are not. Some people also make the mistake of claiming works and skills that they do not own just to make others like them. Avoid the trouble of being shamed when your secrets are discovered. Market your own skills and creations and you would never have to worry about what other people think about you.

Being true to the people whom you are trying to connect with will allow you to maximize the true essence of networking, which is friendship. You will be surprised at how many people are actually willing to accept you and your flaws, and even think that your scars set you apart from the people that they meet. In fact, most of the extremely marketable people are being followed by millions of people because of their humanity.

If you have a human interest story or if you have had a struggle that you were able to survive, then share it to your network. That would show them that you are a person, just like the rest of them. Not only would that make them empathize with you, you are also building additional common ground with them. You are telling them that you are not better than most people, but that you are one of them.

Go Beyond "Be Yourself"

Authenticity will get you to places, help you reach great heights, and most importantly, endear people. However, it is not enough to "be yourself". It is a common error to advise people to simply "be themselves". What if you are not the person you think you want to be? What if you really need to develop and enhance your skills and knowledge, or even your persona?

Instead of simply staying who you are, see to it that you also embrace the persona that you want to be. Do not think about the person that you simply are, but also your potentials. At this point, you are already aware that you do have what it takes to be great, and you are doing all it takes to reach the top, together with the people that you meet. Instead of simply being the person that you are now, make people see your future self – make them feel that they may be talking to a future CEO, or the president. When you embody the greatness that you believe you can achieve, people would push you to reach that goal.

Self-Awareness is Key

Your authenticity lies on the beautiful mix of your battle scars and your beauty – people have always been aware that you have flaws, but will embrace your strengths just the same. By making people aware that you are fine with yourself and that you see that you are a complete package that is still capable of improvement, people would desire to connect with you. They would want to build a relationship with you because you can show that you are human and you can be better.

The secret to being authentic can be unleashed in this way: you should first be self-aware and honest about what you want and who you genuinely are, follow that natural flow of your inner desires and passions, and work towards this. Do not compromise yourself and your passions for a lifestyle that you don't want, for a job you abhor. Do not waste your inner gifts in an environment that does not inspire and motivate you. Otherwise, you will end up looking in the mirror and not knowing who you are in the first place. Lacking self-awareness results to a lack of self-confidence— the ultimate quality that turns people off. This is what you shouldn't be doing to yourself if you want to build relationships, create influence, and strengthen your network.

Be authentic, be who you really are. Not even for others, but ultimately, for yourself. As the saying goes, you can fool others, but you can never lie to yourself. After all, the most essential relationship that you should be building, developing, and cultivating, is the relationship you have with yourself.

Once you nourish this, your colleagues and networks will naturally be endeared to you, finding you likeable, influential, and a unique individual who is prominent in his or her field.

CONCLUSION

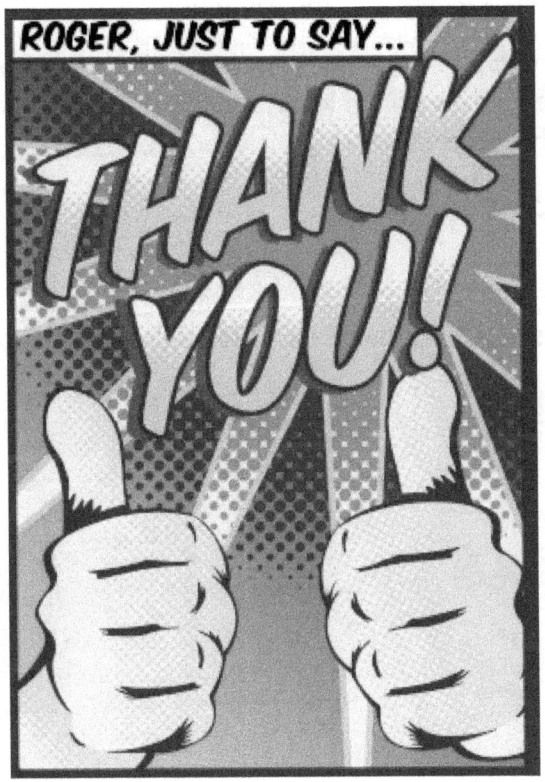

Thank you for reading *Networking: 42 Keys to Career Growth-Communication Skills, Build Relationships, Influence.*

I hope this book left you feeling empowered and armed with the keys that can really and truly unlock endless career growth. Your life, after all, is a huge series of meeting people and connecting with them whether you are trying to get hired or doing the hiring.

The next step is to apply these strategies and remember that this can be the most powerful skill you have, connecting with people. Remember to continue to learn and grow with and from these strategies and see what works for you and your life aspirations.

Finally, if you enjoyed this book, then I'd like to ask you for a favor, would you be kind enough to leave a review for this book on Amazon? It'd be greatly appreciated!

Thank you and good luck!

Don't Forget to Check out Bonus Material at the End of the Book!

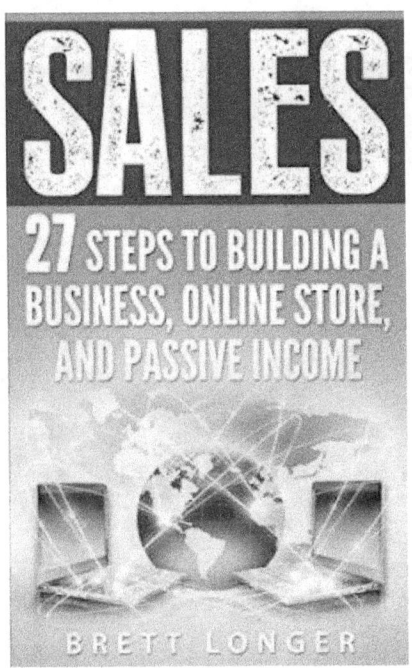

"Organization: The 7 Habits to Organize Your Day, Productivity, and Focus"

When you download *Organization: The 7 Habits to Organize Your Day, Productivity, and Focus*, your quality of life and mindset will transform! You will tap into the methods and habits of the most successful people in the world and what they do on a consistent basis to deliver results.

Available Now on Amazon!

http://amzn.to/1I3BA1K

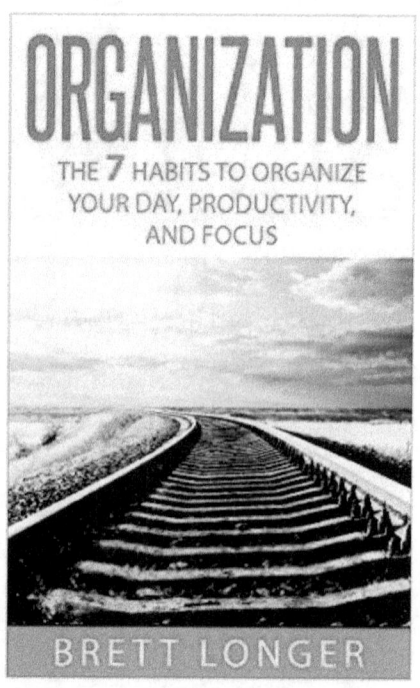

BONUS

The key to networking mostly boils down to if people like you and how to influence them in a way that allows for both of you to win. This bonus is the link to the full audio version of the classic book by Dale Carnegie, "How to Win Friends and Influence People." Listen to it in your car, while you're at home, let the words help you network better through life and see the career growth beyond your wildest dreams.

https://www.youtube.com/watch?v=n4R2p9WnzAol